HEALING HERBS FOR EYE PROBLEMS

The complete natural remedy to get rid of eye Eye problem with mineral, vitamins and powerful herbs from nature

Dr. Gracee Roberts

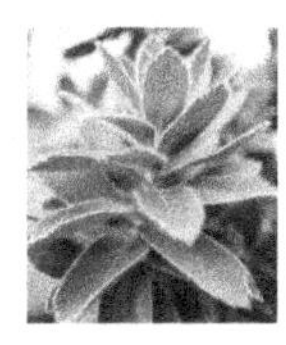
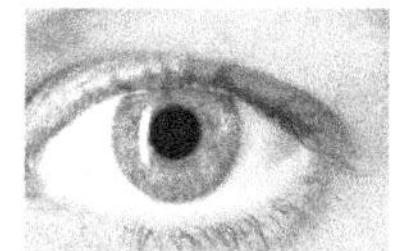

TABLE OF CONTENTS

Introduction

Importance of Natural Remedies

Chapter 1

Understanding Healing Herbs

A. Role of Minerals in Eye Health

B. Essential Vitamins for Eye Care

C. Power of Natural Herbs in Healing

Chapter 2

Common Eye Problems

A. Detailed Explanation of Various Eye Conditions

B. Symptoms and Causes

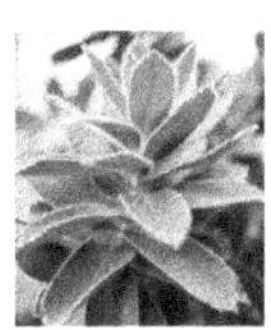
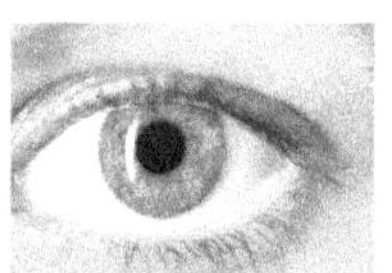

Chapter 3

The Complete Natural Remedy

A. Herbal Solutions for Eye Health

B. Mineral and Vitamin Supplements

C. Creating a Holistic Approach

Chapter 4
Incorporating Nature's Power

A.Integrating Herbs into Daily Life

B. Recipes And Formulas For Eye Health

C. Creating a Holistic Approach

Chapter 5
Lifestyle Tips for Healthy Eyes

A. Nutritional Guidance

B. Eye Exercises and Practices

Chapter 6
Testimonials and Success Stories

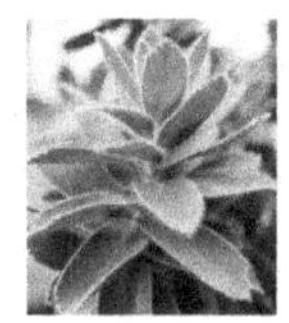 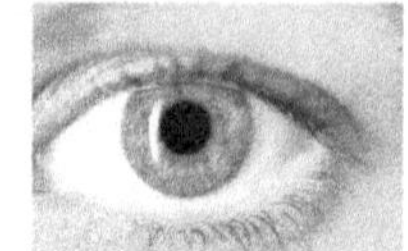

INTRODUCTION

In our fast-paced and technology-driven world, our eyes often bear the brunt of constant strain and exposure to various environmental factors. As a result, eye problems have become increasingly prevalent, affecting individuals of all ages. Recognizing the importance of holistic well-being and the healing potential embedded in nature, "Healing Herbs for Eye Problems: The Complete Natural Remedy" emerges as a comprehensive guide dedicated to alleviating and preventing eye issues through the power of minerals, vitamins, and potent herbs.

This meticulously crafted book looks into the intricate connection between natural remedies and eye health, offering readers a profound understanding of the synergistic effects that minerals, vitamins, and herbs can

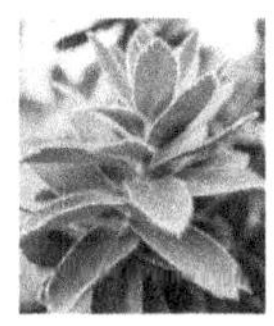

HEALING HERBS FOR EYE PROBLEMS

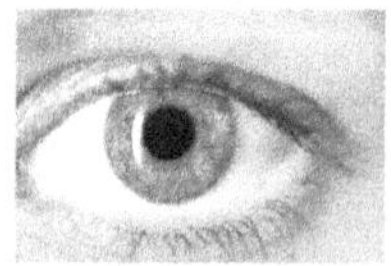

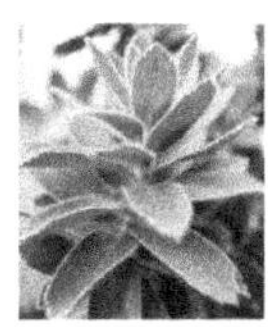
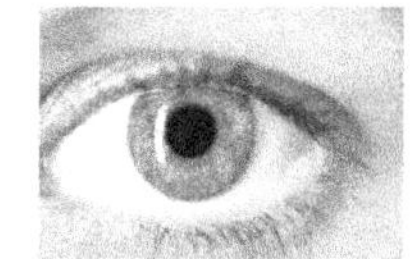

have on promoting optimal vision. The journey begins with an insightful exploration of the common eye problems that plague many, unraveling the complexities behind conditions such as dry eyes, blurred vision, and eye fatigue. By shedding light on the root causes, readers gain invaluable insights into making informed lifestyle choices to safeguard their ocular health.

The heart of this book lies in its meticulous examination of a diverse array of healing herbs sourced directly from nature's pharmacopeia. Each herb is scrutinized for its unique properties, unveiling a treasure trove of remedies that have been revered for centuries in traditional medicine systems. From the soothing embrace of chamomile to the antioxidant-rich prowess of bilberry, the reader is guided through an intricate tapestry of botanical solutions that aim to address specific eye concerns.

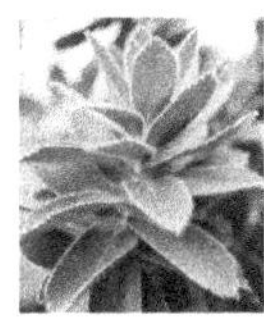
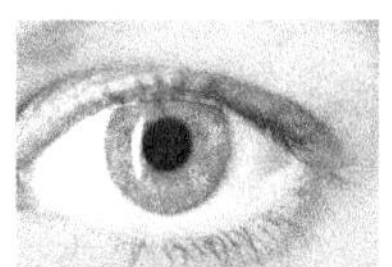

HEALING HERBS FOR EYE PROBLEMS

Furthermore, "Healing Herbs for Eye Problems" empowers readers with knowledge about essential minerals and vitamins crucial for maintaining ocular health. Delving into the science behind nutrients such as vitamin A, C, and E, as well as minerals like zinc and selenium, the book elucidates their roles in supporting vision and fortifying the delicate structures of the eye.

The holistic approach of this guide extends beyond mere identification and understanding, equipping readers with practical strategies for incorporating healing herbs, minerals, and vitamins into their daily lives. Whether through herbal infusions, nutrient-rich recipes, or simple lifestyle adjustments, the book provides a roadmap to seamlessly integrate natural remedies into a busy modern existence.

Embark on a transformative journey towards clearer, healthier vision with "Healing Herbs for Eye Problems." This book transcends conventional approaches, offering a holistic blueprint that celebrates the intricate harmony between nature and ocular well-being. Empower yourself with the knowledge to not only address existing eye issues but to cultivate a proactive and sustainable path towards optimal eye health through the bountiful offerings of minerals, vitamins, and powerful herbs bestowed upon us by nature.

What is is natural remedy

A natural remedy refers to a treatment or solution for health issues that is derived from nature, such as herbs, plants, minerals, or other natural substances. These remedies are often used as alternatives to conventional

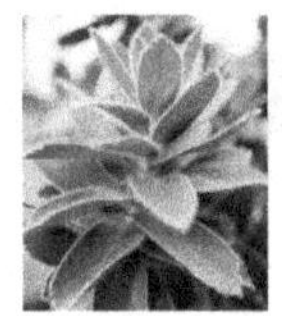 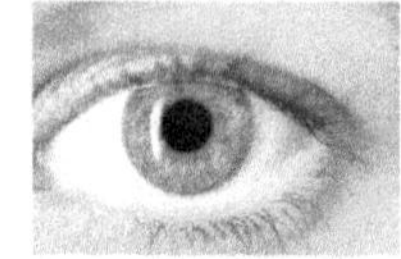

medicine and are believed by some to have healing properties.

Importance of Natural remedies

Natural remedies play a crucial role in promoting holistic health and well-being. Unlike pharmaceutical interventions, which often come with potential side effects, natural remedies harness the healing power of nature without synthetic additives. Here are some key aspects highlighting the importance of natural remedies:

1.Minimal Side Effects: Natural remedies are typically derived from plants, herbs, and other natural sources, minimizing the risk of adverse reactions. This makes them a safer alternative for individuals who may be sensitive or allergic to synthetic compounds found in pharmaceuticals.

2. Holistic Approach: Natural remedies often address the root cause of health issues rather than merely

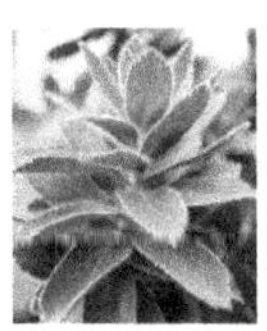 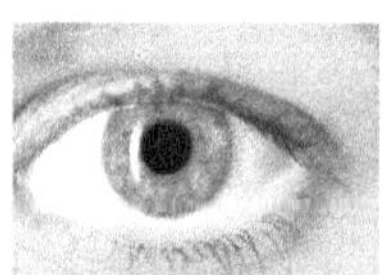

alleviating symptoms. They promote a holistic approach to healing, considering the interconnectedness of various bodily systems and addressing imbalances.

3. Supporting the Body's Innate Healing Abilities: Many natural remedies work by enhancing the body's natural healing mechanisms. For example, herbal teas, essential oils, and certain dietary supplements can boost the immune system, improve digestion, and support overall vitality.

4. Long-Term Health Benefits: Integrating natural remedies into one's lifestyle can contribute to long-term health benefits. Regular consumption of certain herbs, spices, or superfoods may provide ongoing support for various aspects of health, such as cardiovascular function, cognitive health, and stress management.

5. Environmental Sustainability: The cultivation and production of natural remedies often have a lower environmental impact compared to the manufacturing processes involved in pharmaceuticals. This aligns with a growing global emphasis on sustainable and eco-friendly practices.

6. Affordability: Natural remedies are often more cost-effective than prescription medications. This affordability makes them accessible to a broader range of individuals, ensuring that health-promoting practices are not limited by financial constraints.

7. Cultural and Traditional Wisdom: Many natural remedies have been used for centuries in traditional medicine systems around the world. Drawing on the wisdom of these traditions adds a cultural dimension to healing practices, preserving and respecting diverse approaches to well-being.

8. Preventive Health Measures: Natural remedies are frequently employed as preventive measures to maintain overall health. Regular consumption of certain foods, herbs, or supplements can help strengthen the body's defenses and reduce the risk of certain health conditions.

9. Personal Empowerment: Using natural remedies empowers individuals to take an active role in their health. This can involve making informed choices about diet, lifestyle, and self-care practices, fostering a sense of control and responsibility for one's well-being.

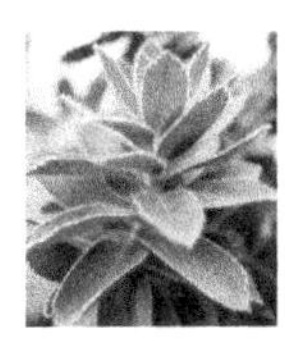
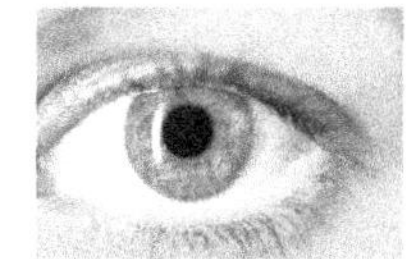

CHAPTER 1

UNDERSTANDING HEALING HERBS

Healing herbs have been utilized for centuries across various cultures for their potential medicinal properties. These plants often contain compounds with therapeutic effects, addressing a wide array of health issues. Understanding healing herbs involves exploring their historical significance, the science behind their efficacy, and practical applications.

Historical Significance:

1.Ancient Remedies: Many traditional healing practices, such as Ayurveda in India or Traditional Chinese Medicine, heavily rely on herbs. These systems date back thousands of years and reflect the accumulated wisdom of generations in using herbs for health.

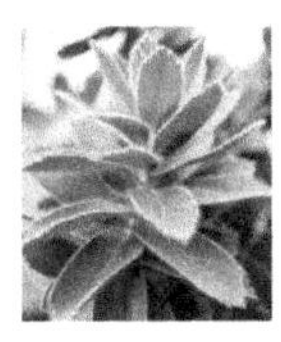

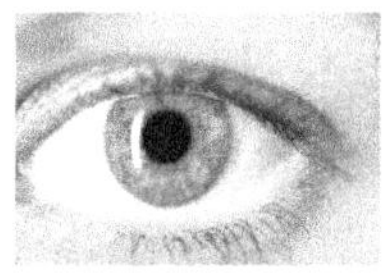

2. Herbalism in Different Cultures: Indigenous cultures worldwide have their own rich traditions of using locally available herbs for medicinal purposes. These practices highlight the intimate connection between communities and their natural surroundings.

Science Behind Healing Herbs

1.Bioactive Compounds: Herbs contain bioactive compounds like alkaloids, flavonoids, and essential oils. These compounds often contribute to the herbs' therapeutic properties by interacting with the human body on a molecular level.

2. Pharmacological Studies: Modern science has delved into the pharmacological aspects of healing herbs. Researchers study how specific compounds influence biological processes, providing a scientific basis for the traditional uses of herbs.

Practical Applications

1.Common Healing Herbs:

Turmeric: Known for its anti-inflammatory properties.

Ginger: Used for digestive issues and nausea.

Echinacea: Believed to boost the immune system.

Lavender: Used for its calming effects.

2. Herbal Remedies:

Teas: Chamomile for relaxation, peppermint for digestion.

Tinctures: Concentrated herbal extracts for specific ailments.

Essential Oils: Extracted from herbs for aromatherapy and topical use.

3. Herbs in Modern Medicine:

Pharmaceuticals: Some drugs trace their origins to herbal compounds, like aspirin from willow bark.

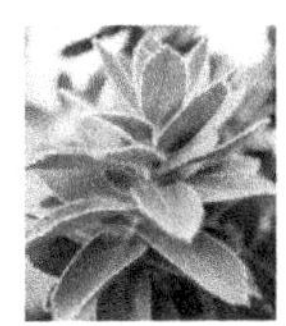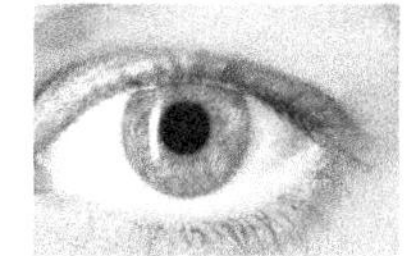

Complementary Medicine: Integrative medicine combines conventional and herbal approaches for holistic health.

Considerations

1.Safety and Dosage:

Not all herbs are safe in all situations; proper dosage is crucial.

Some herbs may interact with medications, emphasizing the importance of consulting healthcare professionals.

2. Cultural and Ethical Considerations:

Respecting traditional knowledge and the cultural significance of certain herbs is vital.

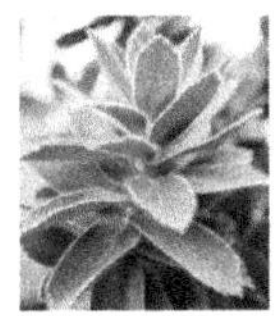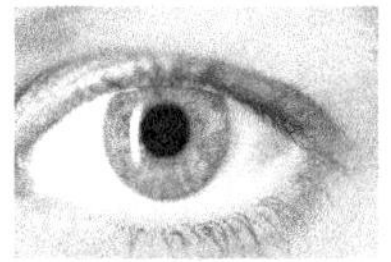

Sustainable harvesting and ethical practices in the herbal industry are increasingly emphasized.

Understanding healing herbs involves recognizing their historical context, the scientific basis of their effects, and their practical applications in diverse cultures and modern healthcare. As with any form of medicine, informed and responsible use is key to harnessing their potential benefits.

Emerging Trends and Research

1.Botanical Medicine Research:

Ongoing studies continue to unveil new therapeutic properties of various herbs.

Research on the synergy of multiple herbs, emphasizing the holistic approach of herbal medicine.

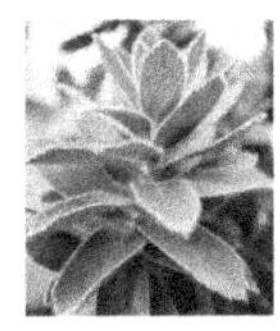 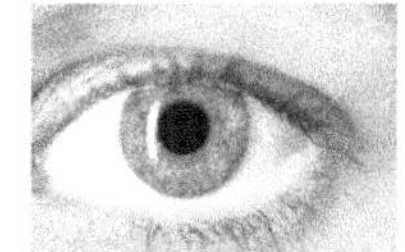

2. Integration with Conventional Medicine:

Growing interest in integrating herbal remedies with conventional medicine for enhanced treatment outcomes.

Recognition of herbs as a valuable source for discovering novel pharmaceuticals.

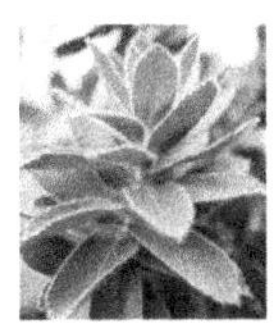 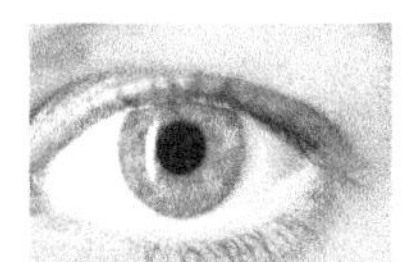

HEALING HERBS FOR EVE PROBLEMS

Popular Healing Herbs and Their Benefits

1.Aloe Vera:

Known for its soothing properties, often used topically for skin conditions.

Contains compounds with potential anti-inflammatory and antioxidant effects.

2.Holy Basil (Tulsi):

Revered in Ayurveda for its adaptogenic properties, helping the body adapt to stress.

Believed to have antimicrobial and anti-inflammatory eeffects.

3. Garlic:

Known for its cardiovascular benefits, including potential blood pressure regulation.

Contains allicin, a compound with antibacterial and antiviral properties.

4.Chamomile:

Popular for its calming effects, often used to alleviate stress and promote sleep.

May have anti-inflammatory properties.

Holistic Healing and Herbalism:

1.Mind-Body Connection:

Herbalism often emphasizes the interconnectedness of physical and mental health.

Certain herbs, like adaptogens, are believed to support overall well-being by helping the body adapt to stress.

2. Holistic Lifestyle Practices:

Herbal remedies are often complemented by lifestyle changes, including nutrition and stress management.

Holistic practitioners focus on addressing root causes rather than just symptoms.

DIY Herbalism and Home Remedies:

1.Growing Interest:

Many individuals are exploring home cultivation of medicinal herbs.

DIY herbalism involves creating teas, tinctures, and salves for personal use.

2. Educational Resources:

Online platforms and books provide information on identifying, cultivating, and using healing herbs.

Workshops and courses on herbalism contribute to the democratization of herbal knowledge.

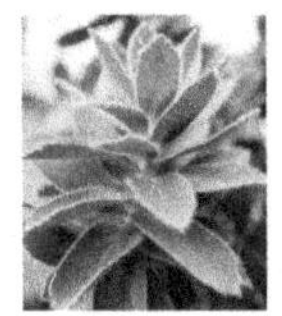 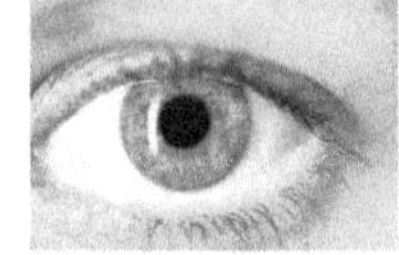

Challenges and Considerations:

1.Quality Control:

Ensuring the purity and quality of herbal products can be challenging.

Standardization of herbal preparations is an ongoing concern.

2. Cultural Appropriation:

With the rising popularity of herbalism, there's a need to address issues of cultural appropriation and respect for traditional knowledge.

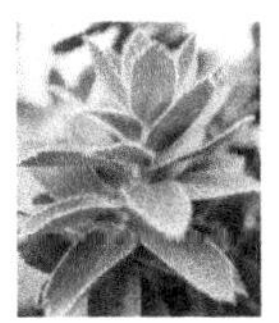

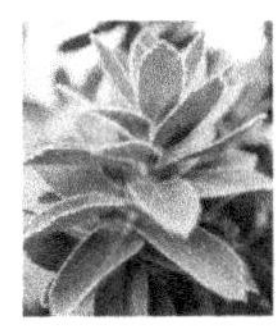
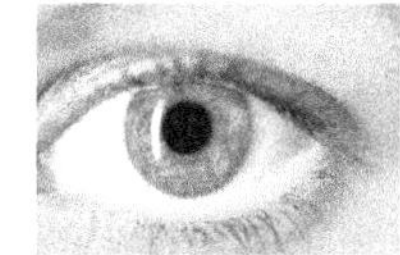

3. Regulatory Framework:

Herbal products face diverse regulatory landscapes globally, highlighting the need for standardized guidelines.

Understanding healing herbs encompasses not only their historical use and scientific underpinnings but also the evolving landscape of herbal medicine in contemporary society. As research continues and cultural awareness grows, the integration of herbalism into holistic healthcare practices is likely to expand, offering diverse options for individuals seeking natural and complementary approaches to well-being.

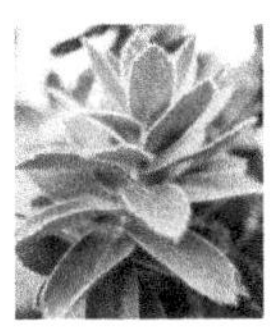
HEALING HERBS FOR EYE PROBLEMS
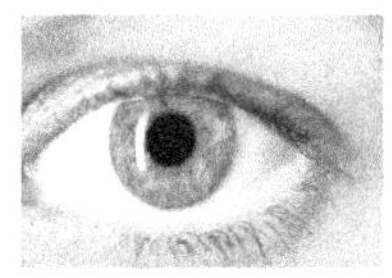

1.1 ROLE OF MINERALS IN EYE HEALTH

Minerals play a crucial role in maintaining optimal eye health, contributing to various functions that support vision and overall well-being. Here's an extensive look at the role of minerals in eye health:

ZINC:

Function: Zinc is essential for the functioning of enzymes involved in maintaining the structural integrity of the eye, particularly the retina. It also supports the transportation of vitamin A from the liver to the retina.

Impact on Eye Health: Zinc deficiency can lead to night blindness and other vision impairments.

COPPER:

Function: Copper is involved in the formation of melanin, a pigment that protects the eyes from ultraviolet (UV) light damage. It also plays a role in the maintenance of connective tissues in the eye.

Impact on Eye Health: Copper deficiency may result in the degeneration of the optic nerve and increased susceptibility to ocular infections.

SELENIUM:

Function: Selenium acts as an antioxidant, protecting the eyes from oxidative stress. It also supports the absorption of vitamin E, which is crucial for maintaining eye health.

Impact on Eye Health: Selenium deficiency may contribute to cataracts and other age-related eye disorders.

MAGNESIUM:

Function: Magnesium is involved in maintaining blood flow to the eyes and regulating intraocular pressure. It also supports the health of blood vessels in the eyes.

Impact on Eye Health: Inadequate magnesium levels may contribute to conditions like glaucoma and retinopathy.

VITAMIN A (RETINOL):

Function: While technically a vitamin, vitamin A is crucial for vision and is often associated with minerals like zinc for optimal absorption.

Impact on Eye Health: Vitamin A deficiency can lead to night blindness and a higher risk of corneal damage.

CALCIUM:

Function: Calcium is essential for the communication between nerve cells, including those involved in transmitting visual information from the eyes to the brain.

Impact on Eye Health: Calcium imbalance may contribute to conditions affecting the optic nerve and visual processing.

POTASSIUM:

Function: Potassium helps regulate fluid balance in the eyes, contributing to the maintenance of proper intraocular pressure.

Impact on Eye Health: Imbalances in potassium levels may lead to increased intraocular pressure, potentially contributing to conditions like glaucoma.

In summary, minerals play a multifaceted role in maintaining eye health, supporting functions ranging from antioxidant protection to structural integrity. A balanced diet rich in minerals, along with vitamins and other nutrients, is crucial for preserving vision and preventing eye-related disorders. Regular eye check-ups and consultation with healthcare professionals are also vital for early detection and management of potential issues.

1.2 ESSENTIAL VITAMINS FOR EYE CARE

Maintaining good eye health is crucial, and certain vitamins play a key role in supporting vision. Here are some essential vitamins for eye care:

1. **Vitamin A:** This vitamin is vital for maintaining the health of the cornea, the outermost layer of the eye. It also plays a crucial role in low-light vision. Foods rich in vitamin A include carrots, sweet potatoes, spinach, and kale.

2. Vitamin E: An antioxidant, vitamin E helps protect cells from damage caused by free radicals. It is found in nuts, seeds, and vegetable oils, contributing to overall eye health.
3. Vitamin C: Known for its immune-boosting properties, vitamin C also supports blood vessels in the eyes. Citrus fruits, strawberries, and bell peppers are excellent sources of this vitamin.
4. Vitamin D: Recent studies suggest a potential link between vitamin D deficiency and age-related macular degeneration (AMD). Fatty fish, fortified dairy products, and exposure to sunlight are good sources of vitamin D.
5. Vitamin B complex (B6, B9, B12): These vitamins contribute to the reduction of inflammation and the prevention of conditions like macular degeneration. Foods like fish, poultry, and leafy greens contain these B vitamins.
6. Zinc: While not a vitamin, zinc is a crucial mineral for eye health. It helps transport vitamin A from the liver to the retina, and it's found in meat, dairy, and whole grains.
7. Omega-3 Fatty Acids: Essential for overall eye health, omega-3 fatty acids, particularly DHA, are

concentrated in the retina. Fatty fish like salmon, flaxseeds, and walnuts are excellent sources.

8. Lutein and Zeaxanthin: These antioxidants are found in high concentrations in the retina and may help protect against harmful high-energy light waves like ultraviolet rays. Leafy greens such as kale, spinach, and collard greens are rich sources.

9. Beta-Carotene: This precursor to vitamin A is crucial for maintaining healthy vision. Carrots, sweet potatoes, and squash are packed with beta-carotene.

10. Copper: While required in smaller amounts, copper is essential for maintaining the health of the optic nerve. Nuts, seeds, and seafood are good dietary sources.

It's important to note that a balanced diet rich in fruits, vegetables, and whole foods generally supports eye health. Regular eye check-ups are also crucial for early detection and prevention of eye-related issues.

1.3 THE POWER OF NATURAL HERBS IN HEALING

Natural herbs have been utilized for centuries across various cultures for their healing properties. These plants contain a myriad of compounds with therapeutic effects on the human body. One of the key advantages of using natural herbs in healing is their holistic approach, often addressing the root cause of ailments rather than merely alleviating symptoms.

Herbs like echinacea, ginger, and garlic are renowned for their immune-boosting properties. Echinacea, for instance, is believed to stimulate the immune system, helping the body fend off infections. Ginger possesses anti-inflammatory and antioxidant effects, while garlic is known for its antimicrobial properties. These herbs collectively contribute to overall well-being by supporting the body's defense mechanisms.

The power of natural herbs extends beyond physical health to mental and emotional well-being. Herbs such as lavender and chamomile have calming properties, aiding in stress reduction and promoting relaxation. Lavender, in particular, is often used in aromatherapy to alleviate anxiety and improve sleep quality.

Traditional medicine systems, such as Ayurveda and Traditional Chinese Medicine, heavily rely on herbs to restore balance within the body. Ayurvedic herbs like ashwagandha and holy basil are adaptogens, helping the body adapt to stress and maintain equilibrium. Traditional Chinese Medicine incorporates herbs like ginseng and astragalus for enhancing energy and vitality.

Additionally, the use of herbs in alternative medicine is gaining traction due to the desire for natural and sustainable healthcare options. Herbal remedies are often considered gentler on the body with fewer side effects compared to synthetic medications. This makes them an attractive choice for those seeking a more harmonious and personalized approach to healing.

It's crucial to acknowledge that while natural herbs offer promising therapeutic benefits, their efficacy may vary, and consultation with healthcare professionals is advisable, especially in severe medical conditions. The power of natural herbs lies not only in their chemical composition but also in the synergy of the compounds they contain, providing a holistic approach to health and well-being.

CHAPTER 2
COMMON EYE PROBLEMS

There are numerous eye conditions that can affect vision and overall eye health.   of some common eye conditions:

1. **Refractive Errors:**
   - *Myopia (Nearsightedness):* Difficulty seeing distant objects clearly.
   - *Hyperopia (Farsightedness):* Difficulty focusing on close objects.
   - *Astigmatism:* Blurred vision due to irregular shape of the cornea or lens.
2. **Age-Related Macular Degeneration (AMD):**
   - Gradual deterioration of the macula, leading to central vision loss.
   - Divided into dry AMD (gradual) and wet AMD (abrupt due to abnormal blood vessel growth).
3. **Cataracts:**

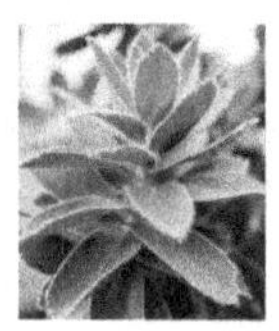 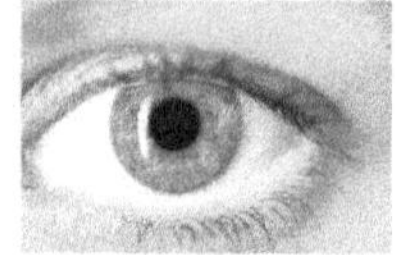

- ○ Clouding of the eye's natural lens, leading to blurred vision.
- ○ Common in aging but can also result from injury or medication.

4. Glaucoma:
- ○ Increased intraocular pressure damaging the optic nerve.
- ○ Gradual peripheral vision loss, often unnoticed until advanced stages.

5. Diabetic Retinopathy:
- ○ Diabetes-related damage to blood vessels in the retina.
- ○ Can lead to vision loss if not managed, with symptoms like floaters and blurred vision.

6. Retinal Detachment:
- ○ Separation of the retina from the underlying tissue.
- ○ Requires immediate medical attention to prevent permanent vision loss.

7. Conjunctivitis (Pink Eye):
- ○ Inflammation of the conjunctiva, causing redness, itching, and discharge.
- ○ Can be infectious or allergic.

8. Keratitis:

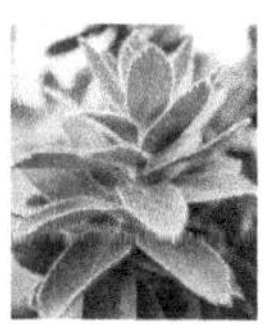 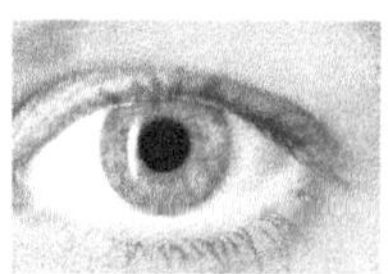

- Inflammation of the cornea often caused by infection or injury.
- Symptoms include pain, redness, and light sensitivity.

9. Strabismus:

- Misalignment of the eyes, affecting binocular vision.
- Can lead to amblyopia (lazy eye) if not treated early in childhood.

10. Ptosis:

- Drooping of the upper eyelid due to weakened muscles.
- Can obstruct vision and may be congenital or acquired.

11. Dry Eye Syndrome:

- Insufficient tear production or poor-quality tears.
- Causes discomfort, redness, and can lead to corneal damage.

12. Color Blindness:

- Inability to perceive certain colors due to genetic factors.
- Most commonly affects the ability to distinguish between red and green.

Understanding these conditions is crucial for early detection and appropriate management. Regular eye exams, lifestyle adjustments, and prompt medical attention can contribute to maintaining good eye health. If you have specific questions about a particular eye condition, feel free to ask!

2.2 Symptoms and Causes of various eye problems

1. **Myopia (Nearsightedness):**
   - *Symptoms:* Blurred distant vision, eye strain.
   - *Causes:* Genetics, excessive screen time, prolonged close-up work.
2. **Hyperopia (Farsightedness):**
   - *Symptoms:* Difficulty focusing on close objects, eye strain.
   - *Causes:* Genetics, aging, certain medical conditions.
3. **Astigmatism:**

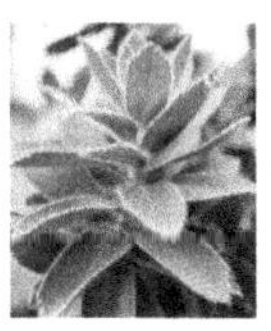
HEALING HERBS FOR EYE PROBLEMS
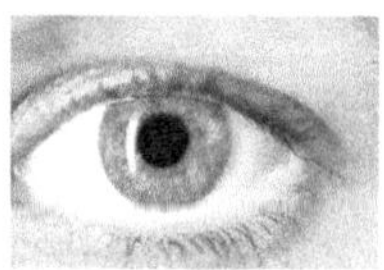

- *Symptoms:* Blurred or distorted vision at all distances, eye discomfort.
- *Causes:* Irregular shape of the cornea or lens, often present from birth.

4. **Presbyopia:**
   - *Symptoms:* Difficulty focusing on close objects, usually noticed with age.
   - *Causes:* Aging, loss of flexibility in the lens.

5. **Cataracts:**
   - *Symptoms:* Cloudy or blurry vision, sensitivity to light.
   - *Causes:* Aging, trauma, certain medications, genetic factors leading to clouding of the eye's lens.

6. **Glaucoma:**
   - *Symptoms:* Gradual loss of peripheral vision, eye pain, headache.
   - *Causes:* Increased intraocular pressure, family history, age.

7. **Macular Degeneration:**
   - *Symptoms:* Central vision loss, distorted vision.
   - *Causes:* Aging, genetics, smoking, high blood pressure.

8. **Conjunctivitis (Pink Eye):**

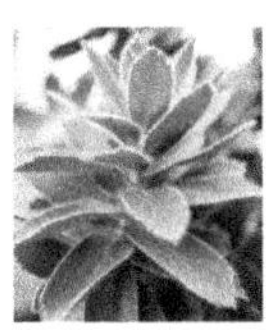 HEALING HERBS FOR EYE PROBLEMS 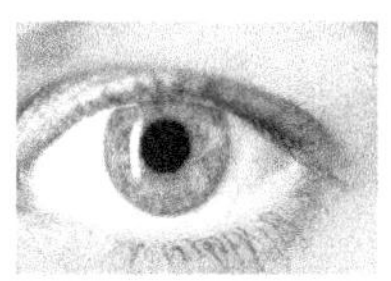

- ○ *Symptoms:* Redness, itching, discharge.
- ○ *Causes:* Viral or bacterial infection, allergies, irritants.

9. **Dry Eye Syndrome:**
- ○ *Symptoms:* Dryness, burning, blurred vision.
- ○ *Causes:* Aging, environmental factors, certain medications.

10. **Retinal Detachment:**
- ○ *Symptoms:* Flashes of light, floaters, sudden vision loss.
- ○ *Causes:* Aging, trauma, family history.

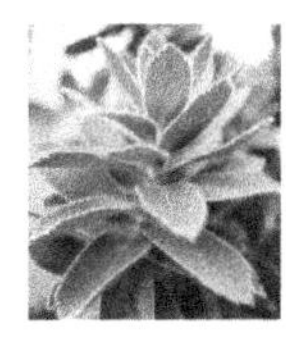
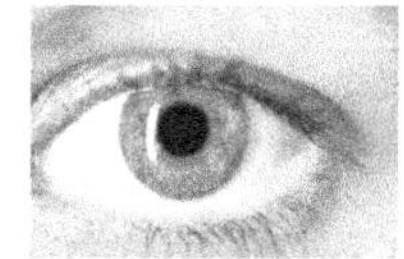

CHAPTER 3

THE COMPLETE NATURAL REMEDY

The health of our eyes is crucial for overall well-being, and incorporating natural remedies can be beneficial in supporting eye health. Several factors, including age, lifestyle, and environmental conditions, can impact our eyes.

Natural remedies for maintaining healthy eyes

Includes

1. **Nutrient-Rich Diet:**
   - Consume foods rich in vitamins A, C, and E, as well as minerals like zinc and selenium. These nutrients play a vital role in maintaining good eyesight.
   - Include leafy greens, carrots, sweet potatoes, citrus fruits, nuts, and seeds in your diet.
2. **Omega-3 Fatty Acids:**

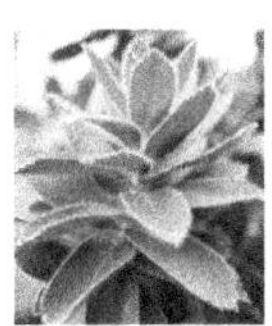
HEALING HERBS FOR EYE PROBLEMS
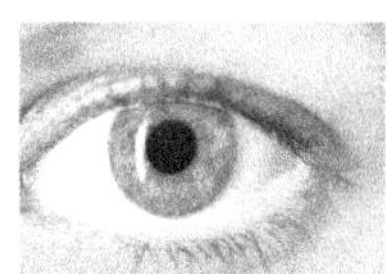

- Incorporate sources of omega-3 fatty acids, such as fatty fish (salmon, mackerel), flaxseeds, and walnuts. These essential fats contribute to the health of the retina.

3. **Stay Hydrated:**
   - Proper hydration is crucial for eye health. Drink an adequate amount of water to prevent dry eyes and maintain overall hydration levels.

4. **Eye Exercises:**
   - Practice eye exercises to relieve eye strain and improve focus. Techniques like the 20-20-20 rule (take a 20-second break every 20 minutes, looking at something 20 feet away) can reduce eye fatigue.

5. **Adequate Sleep:**
   - Ensure you get enough quality sleep to allow your eyes to rest and rejuvenate. Lack of sleep can lead to eye fatigue and dryness.

6. **Herbal Eyewashes:**
   - Utilize herbal infusions like chamomile or calendula for gentle eye washes. These can help soothe irritated eyes and reduce inflammation.

   -

7. **Blinking Exercises:**
   - Perform blinking exercises regularly to keep the eyes moist and prevent dryness. Blinking helps distribute tears, which are essential for eye lubrication.

8. **Reduce Screen Time:**
   - Limit prolonged exposure to digital screens. The blue light emitted from screens can contribute to eye strain. Use blue light filters or take breaks to minimize the impact.

9. **Cold Compress:**
   - Apply a cold compress to reduce eye puffiness and soothe irritation. This can be especially helpful for tired or strained eyes.

10. **Avoid Smoking:**
    - Smoking can increase the risk of developing age-related macular degeneration and other eye conditions. Quitting smoking can positively impact overall eye health.

11. **Maintain Healthy Blood Sugar Levels**:
    - High blood sugar levels can affect the blood vessels in the eyes. Manage your diet to keep blood sugar within a healthy range.

12. **Regular Eye Checkups:**

- Schedule regular eye exams to monitor your eye health and detect any potential issues early on. Professional advice is crucial for maintaining optimal eye care.

3.2 HERBAL SOLUTIONS FOR EYE HEALTH

Herbal solutions for eye health have gained popularity as people seek alternative and natural approaches to maintaining good vision. Several herbs are believed to promote eye health, and they include

1.Bilberry (Vaccinium myrtillus):

Rich in antioxidants called anthocyanins, bilberry is often associated with improving night vision and reducing eye fatigue.

Some studies suggest that bilberry may enhance blood flow to the eyes and protect against oxidative stress.

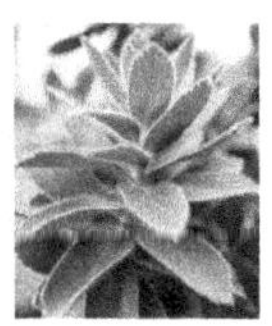
HEALING HERBS FOR EYE PROBLEMS
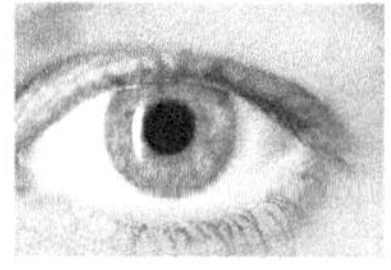

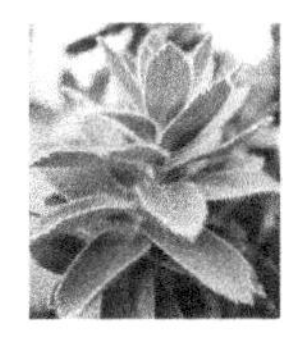

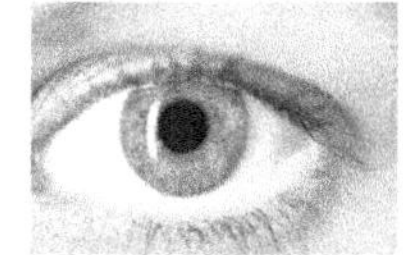

2. Ginkgo Biloba:

Known for its cognitive benefits, ginkgo biloba is also believed to support eye health by improving blood circulation.

Its antioxidant properties may help protect the retina from damage caused by free radicals.

3. Eyebright (Euphrasia officinalis):

Traditionally used in herbal medicine for various eye conditions, eyebright is believed to alleviate eye irritation and inflammation.

It's often used topically as an eyewash or taken orally in tincture or capsule form.

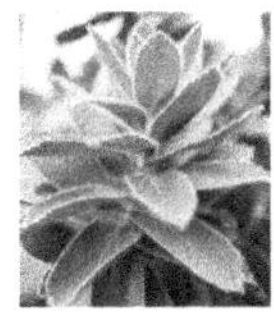

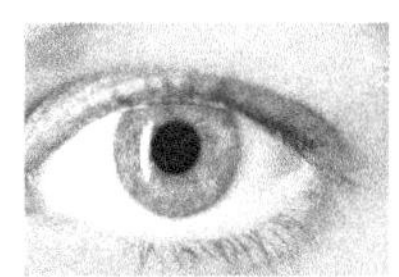

4. Turmeric (Curcuma longa):

Curcumin, the active compound in turmeric, possesses anti-inflammatory and antioxidant properties.

Turmeric may help in managing conditions like uveitis and conjunctivitis, reducing inflammation in the eyes.

5.Fennel (Foeniculum vulgare):

Fennel seeds are rich in nutrients like vitamin C, which is beneficial for eye health.

Some traditional medicine practices suggest fennel infusion as an eye-cleansing remedy.

6. Green Tea (Camellia sinensis):

Green tea is known for its high concentration of antioxidants, including catechins.

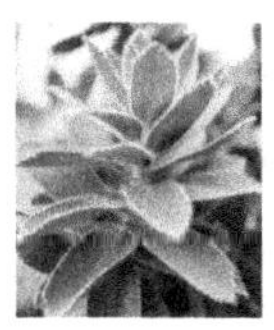 HEALING HERBS FOR EYE PROBLEMS 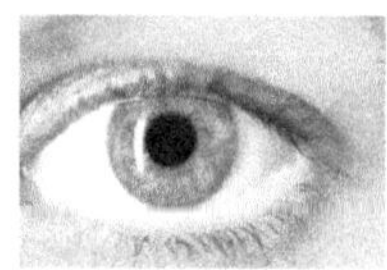

Studies suggest that the antioxidants in green tea may help protect the eyes from age-related diseases.

7. Marigold (Calendula officinalis):

Marigold petals contain lutein and zeaxanthin, carotenoids beneficial for the eyes.

These compounds are believed to protect the eyes from harmful high-energy light waves like ultraviolet rays.

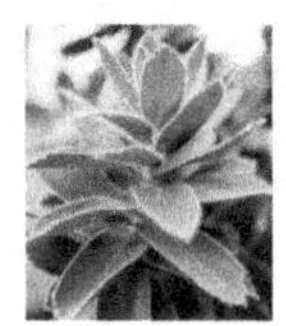 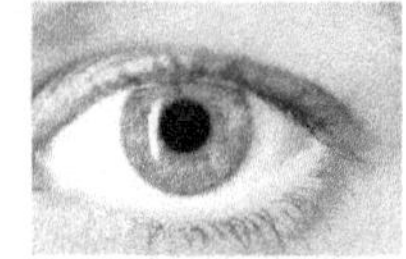

3.3 MINERAL AND VITAMIN SUPPLEMENTS FOR EYE HEALTH

Maintaining good eye health is crucial for overall well-being, and mineral and vitamin supplements can play a significant role in supporting and preserving vision. Several nutrients are particularly essential for eye health, including vitamins A, C, and E, as well as minerals like zinc and selenium.

Vitamin A is a key player in maintaining the health of the cornea, the transparent front part of the eye. It is essential for low-light and color vision. A deficiency in vitamin A can lead to night blindness and other vision impairments. Foods rich in vitamin A include carrots, sweet potatoes, spinach, and eggs.

Vitamin C, known for its antioxidant properties, is crucial for protecting the eyes from oxidative damage caused by

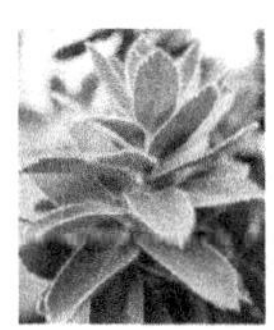 HEALING HERBS FOR EYE PROBLEMS 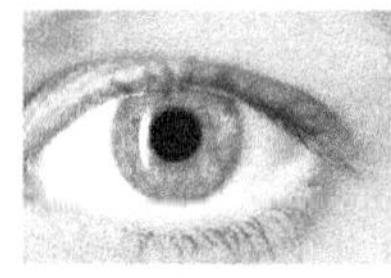

free radicals. Additionally, it supports the health of blood vessels in the eyes. Citrus fruits, strawberries, and bell peppers are excellent sources of vitamin C.

Vitamin E, another powerful antioxidant, helps protect cells, including those in the eyes, from damage. It works in conjunction with vitamin C to maintain eye health. Nuts, seeds, and vegetable oils are good sources of vitamin E.

Zinc is a mineral that is highly concentrated in the eyes, particularly in the retina. It plays a crucial role in maintaining the structure of the eye and is involved in the process of transporting vitamin A from the liver to the retina. Oysters, beef, and pumpkin seeds are rich sources of zinc.

Selenium, another essential mineral, is involved in the production of antioxidant enzymes that help protect the eyes from oxidative stress. Brazil nuts, fish, and whole grains are good dietary sources of selenium.

While a balanced diet that includes these nutrients is essential, some individuals may benefit from supplements to meet their specific needs. However, it's crucial to consult with a healthcare professional before starting any supplement regimen, as excessive intake of certain vitamins and minerals can have adverse effects.

It's worth noting that a healthy lifestyle, including regular eye check-ups, protecting your eyes from harmful UV rays, and avoiding smoking, is fundamental for maintaining optimal eye health. In conclusion, a combination of a nutrient-rich diet, supplements when

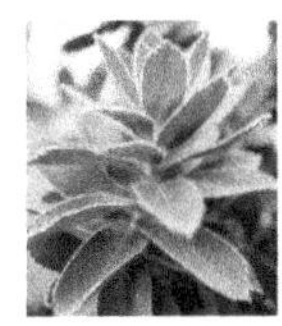
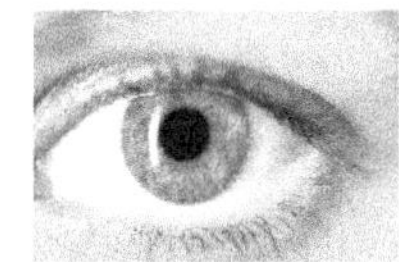

necessary, and lifestyle choices can contribute to the long-term well-being of your eyes.

3.4 CREATING A HOLISTIC APPROACH FOR EYE HEALTH

A holistic approach to eye health involves considering various factors that contribute to overall well-being, incorporating lifestyle choices, nutrition, and regular eye care practices. Here are key aspects to consider:

1. **Nutrition:**
   - Include a balanced diet rich in vitamins and minerals like vitamin A, C, E, and zinc.
   - Omega-3 fatty acids found in fish, flaxseed, and walnuts can promote healthy vision.
2. **Hydration:**
   - Ensure adequate water intake to maintain overall health, including eye moisture.
3. **Eye Exercises:**

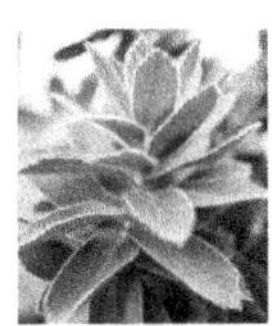
HEALING HERBS FOR EYE PROBLEMS
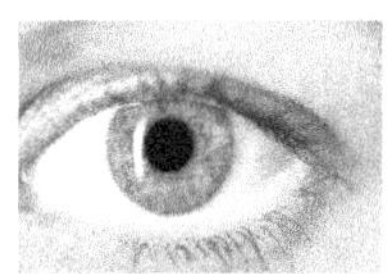

- Practice eye exercises to reduce eye strain, such as the 20-20-20 rule (every 20 minutes, look at something 20 feet away for at least 20 seconds).

4. **Regular Eye Check-ups:**
   - Schedule comprehensive eye exams to detect and address potential issues early on, even if you don't currently wear glasses.

5. **Sleep Hygiene:**
   - Prioritize sufficient and quality sleep to allow your eyes to rest and rejuvenate.

6. **Protective Measures:**
   - Wear sunglasses that block harmful UV rays to prevent cataracts and other UV-related eye conditions.
   - Use protective eyewear in situations where there is a risk of eye injury.

7. **Digital Eye Strain Management:**
   - Follow the 20-20-20 rule when using digital devices extensively.
   - Adjust screen brightness, use anti-glare filters, and maintain proper posture.

8. **Stress Management:**
   - Chronic stress can impact eye health. Incorporate stress-reducing activities like meditation or yoga into your routine.
9. **Environmental Considerations:**
   - Maintain a clean and dust-free environment to reduce the risk of eye irritations and infections.
10. **Holistic Health Practices:**
    - Address underlying health issues like diabetes and hypertension, as they can affect eye health.
    - Consider complementary therapies like acupuncture or acupressure, known for promoting overall wellness.
11. **Limiting Harmful Habits:**
    - Avoid smoking, as it can increase the risk of age-related macular degeneration and other eye conditions.
12. **Educational Outreach:**
    - Promote awareness about eye health in the community to encourage preventive measures and timely interventions.

By integrating these elements into your lifestyle, you can foster a holistic approach to eye health, promoting not just visual acuity but overall well-being for your eyes. Regular self-care, coupled with professional guidance, can significantly contribute to maintaining optimal eye health throughout life.

CHAPTER 4

4.1 INCORPORATING NATURE'S POWER INTO OUR DAILY LIVES

Incorporating nature's power into our daily lives and various aspects of society can bring about numerous benefits, both for the environment and our well-being. One significant way to harness nature's power is through renewable energy sources. Solar power, for instance, taps into the sun's abundant energy, providing a sustainable and clean alternative to traditional fossil fuels. This not only reduces our carbon footprint but also helps combat climate change.

Additionally, wind energy harnesses the power of the wind to generate electricity. Wind turbines are becoming increasingly common, offering a cost-effective and eco-friendly solution. By embracing these renewable sources, we move towards a more sustainable energy future, reducing our dependence on finite resources and minimizing environmental impact.

Beyond energy, incorporating nature's power involves creating green spaces within urban environments. Urban planning that integrates parks, gardens, and trees not only enhances the aesthetic appeal but also improves air quality, mitigates the urban heat island effect, and promotes overall well-being. Access to natural environments within cities has been linked to lower stress levels, increased physical activity, and improved mental health.

Agriculture can also benefit from working in harmony with nature. Practices like agroforestry, permaculture, and organic farming prioritize sustainable and natural methods. These approaches aim to enhance soil health, conserve water, and reduce the need for synthetic pesticides and fertilizers. By adopting nature-inspired agricultural practices, we can create a more resilient and ecologically balanced food system.

Furthermore, biomimicry is a fascinating field that draws inspiration from nature's designs and processes to solve human challenges. Engineers and designers are increasingly looking to natural systems for innovative solutions, whether it's in architecture, material science, or technology. Mimicking the efficiency and elegance of natural processes can lead to breakthroughs in sustainability and resource utilization.

In the realm of healthcare, nature has been recognized for its therapeutic benefits. The concept of "biophilia" suggests that humans have an innate connection with nature and that incorporating natural elements into healthcare settings can contribute to healing and well-being. Hospitals with green spaces, natural light, and views of nature have been shown to positively impact patient recovery rates.

In conclusion, incorporating nature's power extends far beyond a single facet of our lives. It involves a holistic approach that embraces renewable energy, green urban planning, sustainable agriculture, biomimicry, and biophilic design. By recognizing and respecting the inherent power of nature, we can create a more harmonious and sustainable future for generations to come.

4.2 "INTEGRATING HERBS INTO DAILY LIFE

Integrating herbs into daily life can enhance overall well-being by providing numerous health benefits. Incorporating herbs into your routine can be done in various ways, from culinary uses to herbal teas and medicinal applications.

1. Culinary Uses:

Herbs add depth and flavor to your meals, transforming ordinary dishes into culinary delights. Basil, thyme, rosemary, and cilantro are just a few examples of herbs that can elevate the taste of your favorite recipes. Experimenting with different combinations can make your meals not only delicious but also nutritious.

2. Herbal Teas:

Sipping on herbal teas is a soothing way to include herbs in your daily routine. Chamomile, peppermint, and ginger teas are popular choices known for their calming and digestive properties. These teas can be enjoyed throughout the day, providing a natural and gentle boost to your overall well-being.

3. Medicinal Applications:

Many herbs have been traditionally used for their medicinal properties. For instance, turmeric has anti-inflammatory benefits, while lavender is renowned for its calming effects. Incorporating such herbs into your daily routine can contribute to a holistic approach to health, potentially addressing various ailments and promoting overall wellness.

4. Aromatherapy:

Herbs also play a crucial role in aromatherapy, impacting mood and relaxation. Essential oils derived from herbs like lavender, eucalyptus, and peppermint can be diffused or applied topically to promote mental clarity, ease stress, and enhance focus.

5. Home Remedies:

Herbs can be used in simple home remedies to address common ailments. For instance, ginger and honey concoctions for sore throats or aloe vera for skin irritations. Learning about the healing properties of different herbs empowers individuals to address minor health concerns naturally.

6. Gardening:

Growing your own herbs at home not only ensures a fresh supply but also connects you with nature. Whether you have a garden or a small balcony, cultivating herbs like basil, mint, and parsley is a rewarding and sustainable way to integrate them into your daily life.

7. Mindfulness Practices:

Incorporating herbs can become a mindful practice. Taking the time to prepare and savor herbal teas, or cultivating and caring for your herb garden, can be meditative, promoting a sense of calm and connection with nature.

8. Herbal Supplements:

For those seeking a more convenient way to integrate herbs into their routine, herbal supplements provide a concentrated form of beneficial compounds. However, it's essential to consult with a healthcare professional before incorporating supplements to ensure safety and proper dosage.

9. Beauty and Skincare:

Herbs have been used for centuries in beauty and skincare routines. Incorporating herbs like chamomile, aloe vera, or calendula into DIY face masks or skincare products can promote healthy skin and address various skin concerns naturally.

10. Seasonal Rotation:

Consider rotating herbs based on the seasons to align with nature's cycles. For example, focus on warming herbs like ginger and cinnamon during colder months and cooling herbs like mint and cilantro during warmer seasons. This approach not only provides variety but also supports the body's adaptability to different environmental influences.

11. Herbal Education:

Take the time to educate yourself about the properties and uses of different herbs. Understanding the benefits and potential interactions can empower you to make informed choices in integrating herbs into your daily life, ensuring a safe and effective experience.

12. Herbal Workshops and Classes:

Participating in herbal workshops or classes can deepen your knowledge and skills. These opportunities provide hands-on experiences, allowing you to explore herbalism, learn about various herbs, and understand how to incorporate them effectively into your lifestyle.

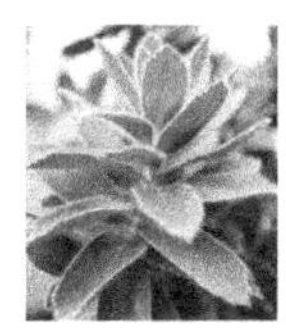
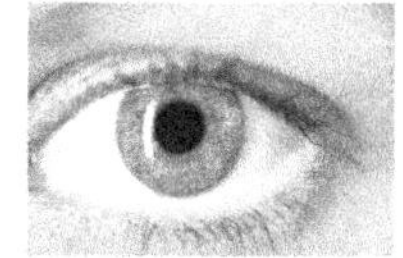

13. Collaborate with Experts:

Engaging with herbalists or holistic health practitioners can offer personalized guidance. They can help tailor herbal recommendations based on your specific health goals, ensuring a more targeted and effective integration of herbs into your daily routine.

14. Family and Community Involvement:

Make herb integration a family or community affair. Cooking with herbs, creating herbal remedies, or maintaining a community herb garden fosters a shared sense of well-being and strengthens social connections.

15. Sustainable Practices:

Embrace sustainable practices by choosing organic and ethically sourced herbs. This not only supports environmental conservation but also ensures the quality

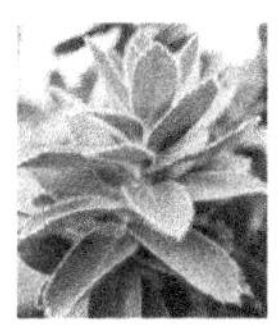
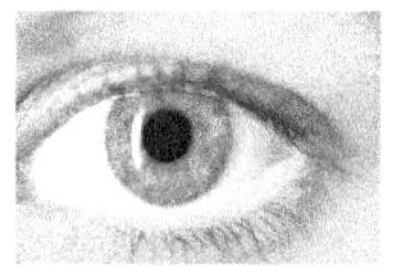

and potency of the herbs you incorporate into your daily life.

By integrating herbs into daily life, individuals have the opportunity to explore a holistic approach to well-being. Whether through culinary delights, herbal teas, medicinal applications, or mindful practices, herbs offer a versatile and natural way to enhance both physical and mental health.

4.4 RECIPES AND FORMULAS FOR EYE HEALTH

I.RECIPE FOR EYE HEALTH

Ingredients:

1.Leafy Greens: Spinach, kale, and collard greens are rich in lutein and zeaxanthin, antioxidants that support eye health.

2. Fatty Fish: Salmon, trout, and sardines contain omega-3 fatty acids, which contribute to the health of the retina.

3. Colorful Fruits and Vegetables: Carrots, sweet potatoes, and bell peppers provide beta-carotene and vitamin A, essential for maintaining vision.

4. Nuts and Seeds: Almonds, walnuts, and chia seeds offer vitamin E and zinc, supporting overall eye health.

5. Citrus Fruits: Oranges, grapefruits, and lemons provide vitamin C, which may reduce the risk of age-related macular degeneration.

6. Eggs: Rich in lutein, zeaxanthin, and zinc, eggs contribute to the prevention of macular degeneration.

7. Whole Grains: Brown rice, quinoa, and whole wheat bread contain vitamin E, zinc, and niacin beneficial for eye health.

II. FORMULAS FOR EYE HEALTH

1.Omega-3 Boost Smoothie: Blend together spinach, kale, a handful of blueberries, a tablespoon of chia seeds, and a portion of fatty fish oil.

2. Antioxidant Salad: Combine mixed greens, carrots, bell peppers, and a sprinkle of sunflower seeds. Drizzle with olive oil for added healthy fats.

3. Citrus Infused Water: Make a refreshing drink with slices of citrus fruits like oranges and lemons in water to stay hydrated and get a vitamin C boboost.

4. Baked Salmon with Veggies: Season salmon fillets with a dash of olive oil, garlic, and lemon. Bake alongside a mix of colorful vegetables like cherry tomatoes, broccoli, and carrots for a nutrient-packed meal.

5. Carrot and Sweet Potato Soup: Create a comforting soup by simmering carrots, sweet potatoes, onions, and a hint of ginger. Blend until smooth for a delicious, vitamin A-rich dish.

6. Almond and Berry Parfait: Layer Greek yogurt with fresh berries and a sprinkle of almonds for a tasty treat that provides a mix of antioxidants, vitamins, and minerals.

7. Egg and Spinach Omelette: Whisk eggs and fold in spinach leaves. Cook with a touch of olive oil for a protein-packed breakfast that supports eye health.

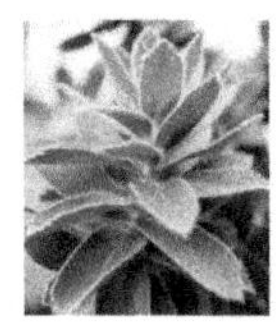

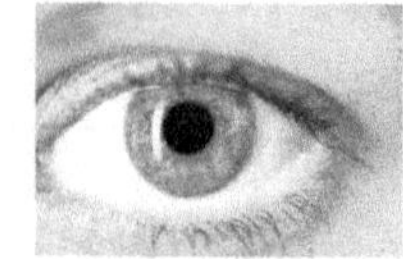

CHAPTER 5

LIFESTYLE TIPS FOR HEALTHY EYES

Maintaining healthy eyes involves adopting a holistic approach to lifestyle choices. Adequate sleep is crucial, as it allows the eyes to rest and regenerate. Additionally, managing stress is essential, as prolonged stress can contribute to eye strain and discomfort.

Regular eye check-ups are vital for early detection of any potential issues. Protecting your eyes from harmful ultraviolet (UV) rays by wearing sunglasses when outdoors can prevent long-term damage. Furthermore, avoiding smoking and limiting alcohol intake can positively impact eye health.

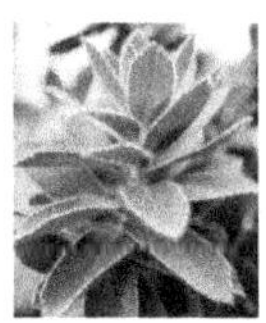

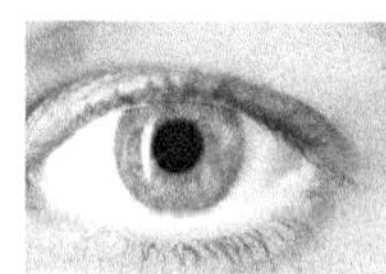

5.1 NUTRITIONAL GUIDANCE FOR HEALTHY EYES

Maintaining good eye health involves a combination of proper nutrition, lifestyle choices, and regular eye care.

1.Vitamins and Minerals:

Vitamin A: Essential for maintaining the health of the retina. Sources include carrots, sweet potatoes, spinach, and eggs.

Vitamin C: Boosts collagen production and helps prevent age-related macular degeneration (AMD). Citrus fruits, strawberries, and bell peppers are rich sources.

Vitamin E: Acts as an antioxidant and protects cells in the eyes. Almonds, sunflower seeds, and spinach are good sources.

2. Omega-3 Fatty Acids:

Found in fish oil, flaxseed, and walnuts, omega-3 fatty acids contribute to the overall health of the eyes. They are particularly beneficial for preventing dry eyes and reducing the risk of AMD.

3. Lutein and Zeaxanthin:

These carotenoids are found in high concentrations in the retina and can help protect against AMD and cataracts. Leafy green vegetables, broccoli, and eggs are excellent sources.

4. Zinc:

Plays a crucial role in transporting vitamin A from the liver to the retina. It is found in meat, dairy products, nuts, and whole grains.

5. Antioxidants:

Foods rich in antioxidants, such as berries, dark chocolate, and green tea, help protect the eyes from oxidative stress and may reduce the risk of developing eye diseases.

6. Hydration:

Staying well-hydrated is essential for overall health, including eye health. Dehydration can lead to dry eyes and discomfort. Aim to drink plenty of water throughout the day.

6. Maintain a Healthy Weight:

Obesity increases the risk of developing diabetes, which in turn can lead to diabetic retinopathy. Maintaining a healthy weight through balanced nutrition and regular exercise is crucial.

7. Limit Sugary and Processed Foods:

Diets high in processed foods and added sugars can contribute to inflammation and increase the risk of developing diabetes, which is a major cause of vision loss.

8. Protective Eyewear:

While not directly related to nutrition, wearing sunglasses that block UV rays can help prevent cataracts and protect the eyes from sun damage.

9. Regular Eye Check-ups:

Schedule regular eye exams to detect any potential issues early on. Comprehensive eye care includes not only nutritional aspécts but also monitoring overall eye health.

5.2 EYE EXERCISES AND PRACTICES

Eye exercises and practices are essential for maintaining good eye health and preventing eye strain, especially in today's digital age where we spend considerable time staring at screens. Here are effective eye exercises and practices:

1.Palming: Rub your hands together to generate warmth, then gently place them over your closed eyes without applying pressure.

Breathe deeply and relax for a few minutes, allowing the warmth to soothe your eyes and relieve tension.

2. 20-20-20 Rule: Follow the 20-20-20 rule to reduce eye strain during prolonged screen time.

Every 20 minutes, look at something 20 feet away for at least 20 seconds to give your eyes a break.

3. Blinking Exercises: Blinking helps to moisten the eyes and prevent dryness. consciously blink every 5-10 seconds when staring at a screen.

4. Eye Rolling: Slowly roll your eyes clockwise, then counterclockwise. This helps improve flexibility and reduces eye stiffness.

5. Focusing: Hold a pen at arm's length and focus on the tip. Slowly bring it closer to your nose, then move it back out. Repeat this several times to improve focus.

6. Near and Far Focus: Choose an object close to you and focus on it for a few seconds, then shift your focus to a distant object. Repeat this process to enhance flexibility in your eye muscles.

7. Eye Massage: Gently massage your temples and the area around your eyes in circular motions with your

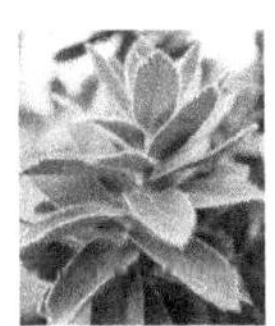 HEALING HERBS FOR EYE PROBLEMS 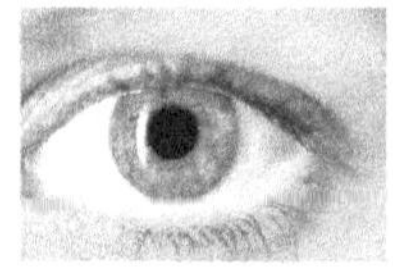

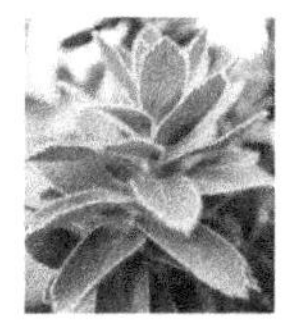
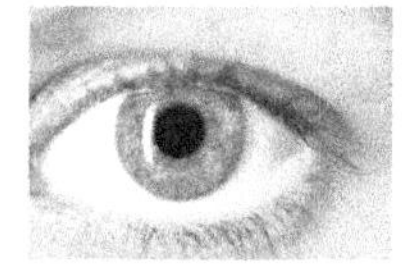

fingertips. This can help alleviate tension and improve blood circulation.

8. Eye Aerobics: Follow eye aerobics routines that involve moving your eyes in different directions – up and down, side to side, diagonally. This improves eye coordination.

9. Visualizing: Close your eyes and visualize a distant scene, such as a calming beach or a peaceful forest. This helps in relaxing your eye muscles.

10. Pencil Push-ups: Hold a pencil at arm's length and focus on the eraser. Slowly bring it towards your nose, maintaining focus. This helps in improving convergence.

11. Eye Yoga: Incorporate yoga poses that involve eye movement, like the "palming" pose or the "trataka" technique, to strengthen eye muscles.

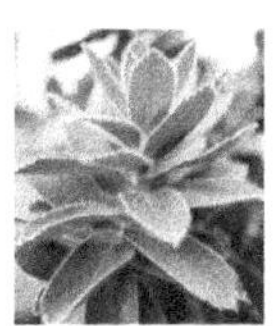
HEALING HERBS FOR EYE PROBLEMS
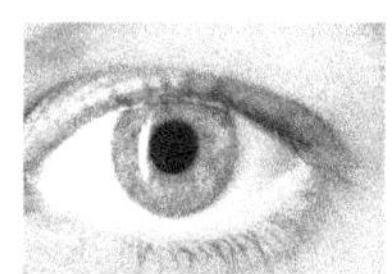

CHAPTER 6
TESTIMONIALS AND SUCCESS STORIES

1.John's Journey to Clear Vision:
After struggling with deteriorating eyesight, John discovered the power of natural remedies for eye health. Through a combination of eye exercises and a nutrient-rich diet, he experienced significant improvements. Now, John enjoys clear vision and a renewed zest for life.

2. Emma's Remarkable Vision Transformation:
Emma, facing challenges with her eyesight, turned to natural remedies. Incorporating antioxidants and omega-3 fatty acids into her daily routine, she witnessed a remarkable improvement. Emma now shares her story to inspire others on their journey to better eye health.

3. David's Struggle with Dry Eyes:
David battled chronic dry eyes for years until he embraced natural remedies. By staying hydrated, using warm compresses, and including foods rich in vitamins A and D in his diet, David found relief. His success story

stands as a testament to the effectiveness of holistic approaches.

4. Sophia's Triumph Over Digital Eye Strain: Constant screen exposure took a toll on Sophia's eyes, causing discomfort and strain. Through regular breaks, eye exercises, and herbal eye drops, she successfully overcame digital eye strain. Sophia now advocates for the importance of mindful eye care in the digital age.

5. Michael's Journey to Combat Age-Related Macular Degeneration (AMD):
Faced with AMD, Michael turned to natural remedies like lutein-rich foods and supplements. Combined with a healthy lifestyle, these interventions slowed the progression of his condition. Michael's perseverance and commitment to natural solutions showcase the potential for managing age-related eye issues.

These testimonials highlight the diverse ways individuals

have incorporated natural remedies into their lives,

leading to positive outcomes in their eye health.

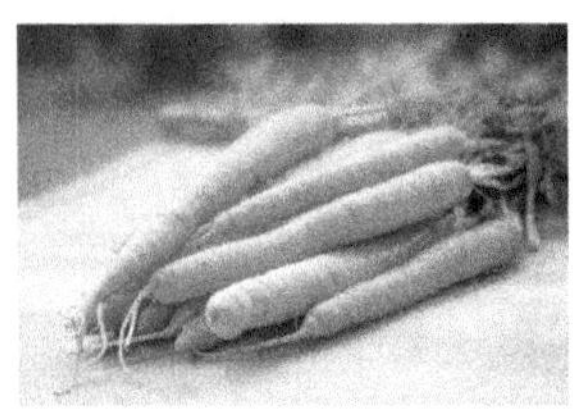

Carrots

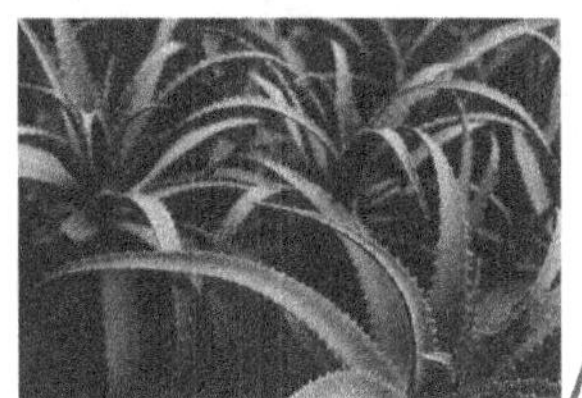

Aloe vera

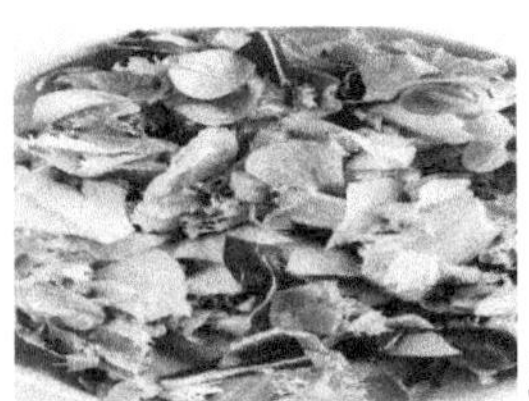

Spinach.

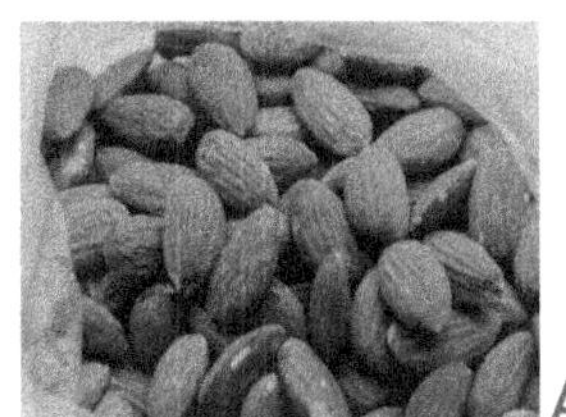

Almond